# Hormone Res

# Meal Plan

## *21 Day Hormone Reset Diet Plan*

**Leona Edward**

# Introduction

When it comes to losing weight, we focus so much on eating the right kind of foods that are nutritious but low in calorie as well as exercising to burn any extra calories. While doing all the above is very important, did you know that you could do all that and not even lose a single pound? Why, you may wonder? Because weight loss is more than just reducing your calorie intake and exercising, actually, your hormones could actually sabotage your weight loss goals.

You may probably be wondering....

How can my hormones affect my weight loss?

What hormones are these?

How can I correct that and achieve my weight loss goals?

Well, all that and more will be covered in this book. In this book, you will learn about the hormone reset diet that enables you to reset key hormones that affect your weight.

By the time you finish reading this book, you will know what you need to do in addition to reducing your calorie intake and working out to lose weight.

# Table of Contents

# Chapter 1: The Hormone Reset Diet Explained

We often overlook how intensely hormones affect our bodily functions, let alone weight loss/gain. Our hormones can determine our stress levels, cause acne, change our mood, as well as affecting our sex drive. A Hormone Reset Diet focuses on making your hormones efficient and boosting your metabolism to ensure constant weight loss.

It does so by resetting the functioning of 7 of the metabolic hormones in the body through a method of eliminating various triggers that cause an imbalance in a bid to resynchronize your metabolism.

The seven hormones include insulin, cortisol, testosterone, leptin, estrogen, thyroid, and growth hormone. How exactly does it achieve that? We will learn that as we discuss how the diet works next.

## How The Diet Works

In addition to weight gain being caused by eating more calories than your body needs, sometimes, it can also be caused by an imbalance of these seven hormones. If you have been trying to lose weight and even significantly limit your calorie intake to achieve weight loss but nothing much happens, then your hormones could be the reason why you still keep on gaining weight and have a difficult time losing it.

When your body does not function as it should and develops some resistance to the hormones, your metabolism slows down and causes your body to store fat every time you eat instead of converting it into energy for use by the body, which significantly leads to gaining of weight while making it quite difficult to lose weight. The hormone reset diet, however, works to reverse this by 'fixing' your 'broken' metabolism.

The hormone reset diet incorporates three-day bursts where you focus on making specific dietary changes in 21 days. Every three days, you cut off particular foods that could be messing up your metabolism and switch to better and healthier foods to bring harmony to your hormones. The diet recommends three days because this is the minimum amount of time that your body requires to reset a hormone. So doing this every three days with each of the seven hormones gives you a total of 21 days to reset all the hormones.

## After Resetting

Once you are done resetting, you will now add back foods that are nutrient-dense one by one, and this process is known as reentry. By consciously listening to your body as you slowly add back the foods, you will be able to note when your hormonal system is triggered and the foods you need to completely avoid or reduce their intake so that your body can function effectively.

### *An Overview Of Hormone Resetting*

When doing your hormone resetting, the following order has been proven to be most effective:

**Meatless-** an essential step that excludes red meat and alcohol and aims at resetting your estrogen

**Sugar-free-** resets your insulin and curbs sugar cravings

**Fruitless-** focuses on resetting leptin- the hunger hormone.

**Caffeine-free-** targets the hormone cortisol and your stress levels.

**Grain-free-** focuses on activating the thyroid hormone intensely and resets leptin and insulin.

**Dairy-free-** targets the growth hormone and improves insulin

**Toxin-free-** this sets your testosterone levels to normal and assists in resetting insulin, thyroid, estrogen and leptin.

After you are done with all these steps, you can now start adding the above foods little by little while listening to your body. If something feels off, then you should avoid it completely or reduce how much of it you eat.

Let us now look at the seven hormones in-depth and learn why it is critical to balance them for effective body functioning and to achieve weight loss.

# Chapter 2: Resetting The Seven Hormones

Remember that you should do these resets for three days for each hormone.

## Meatless: For Resetting Estrogen

Carnivores usually have higher levels of estrogen compared to vegetarians, and this is because of the hormones present in meat. For instance, the hormone estrogen is given to the feedlot cattle (cattle that are fattened for the market) to promote growth. So when you go meatless, the level of estrogen decreases.

Let us learn how estrogen can affect your weight:

### Estrogen And Weight

Estrogen, as a female hormone, has a variety of effects on the body that can promote weight gain. However, this ideally depends on the state of your body. When you are younger and productive, estrogen triggers the storage of fats to ensure fertility, which means weight gain.

Around menopause, one form of estrogen known as estradiol decrease. This hormone is vital in regulating your metabolism and weight. Therefore, reduction in its levels means weight gain.

## Meatless Rules (For The 1st Three Days)

### *(Check on weaning off caffeine before you begin)*

**#1:** Incorporate good and healthy fats. Don't be fooled; good fats won't clog your arteries. There are both good and bad fats; therefore, you should aim to eat unprocessed and natural fats that are found in whole foods. For instance, the best oils for cooking would be organic virgin red palm oil and organic coconut oil. Avoid industrial polyunsaturated fats such as safflower, soybean, cottonseed and corn oil. Other great sources of fats include avocado and nuts.

**#2:** Don't eat meat or drink alcohol (consuming alcohol can increase the levels of estrogen).You should consume not less than a pound of veggies (about 5 to 10 cups depending on the vegetables) each day spread between 3 meals with some healthy proteins.

**#3:** Have your daily fiber intake at around 35 to 45 grams for women and 40 to 50 for men (basically increasing intake by

5g), which will help your liver to clean out the excess estrogen.

## Food List For This Phase

### *Veggies*

Cauliflower, kohlrabi, squash, turnip, bell pepper, radish, broccoli, cabbage, chicory, arugula, watercress, collards, Swiss chard, kale, etc

### *Legumes*

You can also have lentils and all types of beans

### *Nuts*

Nuts and nut butters (e.g., cashew and almond butter) and seeds.

### *Healthy fats*

Coldwater fish are a great source of polyunsaturated fats. Others are crustaceans (crab, shrimp and oysters), evening primrose oil and borage, clarified butter (pastured ghee)

The healthy sources of monounsaturated fats include dark chocolate, avocados, duck fat, Healthy saturated fats come from MCT oil (medium-chain triglycerides) coconut oil and red palm oil.

To increase fiber intake in addition to eating vegetables, consume ground flax seeds, chia seeds, low glycemic fruits such as berries, fiber powders and capsules (which should be added to shakes).

For soy, avoid GM (genetically modified) soy and enjoy whole and fermented soy.

## Sugarless: For Resetting Insulin

You have to cut all kind of sugar from your diet, which means no cookies, soda, cakes, ice cream, and muffins. You have to be a little cautious here and thoroughly look at labels because sugar can hide in not so obvious names; for example, fructose, dextrose, malt syrup, maltose etc.

Let us understand the relationship between insulin and weight:

### Insulin And Weight

Insulin is the hormone that is majorly responsible for the processing of sugars. Increased intake of foods that are broken down into glucose means that your body has to produce more and more insulin to help the cells absorb the glucose with the excess being converted to fat.

When you are always eating foods high in carbohydrates, your body never gets time to tap into your fat stores to burn them for energy because there is always a ready supply of glucose. As long as your insulin levels are always high, your body will not burn fat for energy; hence, constant weight gain.

## Sugar Addiction

The thing about sugar is that it is addictive. Foods high in sugar trigger reward centers in your brain and if you are vulnerable to food addiction, this can be problematic.

The more you eat sugar, the more you develop issues with dopamine communication; hence you need more sugary foods to raise your dopamine and feel 'normal.' To interrupt this pattern, eliminating sugar is essential.

## Sugarless Rules

**#1.** Remove sugar and its substitutes. Avoid honey, agave, white and brown table sugar, Splenda, molasses and maple syrup.

Be aware of hidden sugars in sauces, packaged cereals, dressings, and ketchup. Liquid sugar, including alcohol, soda and diet soda, juice and lemonade, should also be eliminated.

**#2.** Include probiotic foods. Fermented foods with natural probiotics (or healthy bacteria) can dramatically boost your health. They add good bacteria to your stomach and are great for detoxification, especially when it comes to heavy metals. A good example is kimchi which prevents several conditions such as diabetes, yeast infection, UTI's, obesity and gastrointestinal cancers.

**#3.** Eat a pound of veggies- cooked and raw. Keep eating about 3 to 4 cups a day. You can incorporate them into your breakfast (e.g., a salad for breakfast), lunch and dinner quite easily. You can also add them to shakes.

You can try having steamed veggies at hand to add them to your meals. Avoid starchy veggies and stick to vegetables that are dark as they have a low glycemic index and are packed with essential nutrients.

**#4.** Have at least a meal every 4 to 6 hours. If you constantly feel the need to snack and can basically eat anything in about 3 hours, then it's pretty evident that you are insulin resistant and need this reset badly.

If you feel the urge to snack, first try and have some water and wait for about 20 minutes. If you still are hungry after that, have yourself some walnuts, almonds or veggies snacks.

**#5.** Have protein in each meal (about 4 to 6 ounces).

**#6.** Have 1 half cup of low glycemic fruit (an index of 55 or below) such as avocados, olives and berries.

## Food List For This Phase

### *Sugar and carbs*

Go for the slow carbs that won't spike your insulin such as quinoa, yams, pumpkins, sweet potatoes. When it comes to sugar substitutes, you can only use stevia.

### *Vegetables*

These include broccoli, asparagus, mushrooms, red bell peppers, zucchini and arugula. For the leafy green vegetable, go for the darker ones such as kale, dandelion greens, collards, spinach, chard, sweet potato leaves etc.

### *Proteins*

Eat freely, fish (salmon, sardines, mackerel, and cod), chicken (pastured, free-range or organic), eggs, lentils, black beans, white kidney beans, pinto beans.

### *Fruits*

You can eat avocados, coconut, berries and olives.

### *Fermented foods*

These include kefir, fermented veggies such as pickles and sauerkraut, miso, yogurt, fermented milk, and kimchi.

## Fruitless: For Resetting Leptin

Fructose, the sugar found in fruits, is linked to problems with insulin and another hormone known as leptin that is in charge of hunger. When you are full, leptin is produced and communicates with your brain to give you feelings of satiety. Once you experience blood sugar issues and/or you are overweight, fructose can become a problem for this hormone.

Did you know that fructose is 73% sweeter than normal sugar making it highly delectable and promotes overeating? But how much fructose is too much? This majorly depends on your metabolism, genetics, how active/fit you are and what you are eating. 20 grams (or less) of fructose daily is ideal for a reset.

## Leptin And Weight

The liver is the only organ that processes fructose. If you eat a lot of fructose, your liver will not be able to process the fructose fast enough for the body to utilize it as fuel energy. Instead, the body begins converting the fructose into fats and releasing them as triglycerides into the bloodstream or depositing them into the liver and elsewhere on your abdomen as fat. Usually, leptin is produced by fat cells; however, with increased intake of fructose, your fat cells produce excess leptin and the leptin receptors can't be able to keep up with the feedback loop. You would think that more leptin would suppress your appetite but the total opposite happens. When your brain receives too much leptin signals, it shuts down from being overflown.

The result from this: levels of leptin continue rising, receptors don't function (your body doesn't get the leptin signal), you stop feeling full, you keep eating all the wrong foods, which inevitably lead to leptin resistance and weight gain.

The best way to keep leptin under control and to have it work the way it should (now that at this point your insulin is intact) is by cutting back on fructose and consuming more clean protein.

## Fruitless Rules

Follow the following rules to have leptin working with you instead of against you:

**#1.** Your first meal should be protein. Within 30 minutes of waking up, make sure to have some protein to reduce cravings- you can have some eggs. For the rest of the day, have moderate amounts of protein, about 75- 100 grams a day.

**#2.** Quit snacking. Snacking is often a habit reflecting disconnection from real hunger. Resist the urge and have three meals a day and time the meals every 4 to 6 hours. Normal leptin levels will ensure you don't feel hungry in between meals.

**#3.** Have a pound of low fructose vegetables. As much as vegetables are a good source of antioxidants and fiber, they can also contain fructose. The veggies you should eat should contain less than a gram of fructose per 200 calorie serving.

Such veggies include sauerkraut, alfalfa sprouts, peas, spinach and artichokes. Other vegetables such as sweet potatoes, squash, broccoli and carrots can also be consumed as they have less than 5 grams of protein and have high fiber content- as long as the total fructose per day doesn't exceed 20 grams.

**#4.** Cut back on alcohol.

**#5.** Stay away from nightshade veggies and fruits, as these plants can cause inflammation in some people as they contain a chemical known as solanine that can mess up enzymes in the muscles. This can lead to stiffness and pain and cause you some serious digestive problems.

You might be sensitive to such fruits and plants and may have never realized that they may be the cause of your joint discomfort and gut issues. Keep away from nightshades such as eggplant, potatoes, bell peppers, tomatoes, and tomatillos for three days. Also, avoid GMO soy that has been hybridized with petunia, which is a nightshade.

**#6.** Eat healthy fats. Some great sources of fat include coconut oil and coconut, butter, nuts, avocados, and animal fats.

# Caffeine Free: For Resetting Cortisol

Coffee is great if taken in small quantities since high levels of intake can be toxic and lead to a shift of mood, increased anxiety, can mess up your sleep and even lead to palpitations.

So how does coffee affect weight loss?

## Cortisol And Weight

Consuming coffee regularly and in high amounts disrupts your natural circadian rhythm that controls your hormonal harmony. Such a disruption can lead to weight gain because coffee heightens cortisol (commonly known as the stress hormone), which is a crucial hormone in fat storage, regulating metabolism and controlling blood pressure and sugar.

When cortisol is too low or too high, it has its adverse effects on your body either way. Extremely high cortisol levels disrupt your sleep, make you moody and can lead to weight gain. Low levels of cortisol live you feeling suppressed.

### *Weaning yourself off caffeine*

It can be a bit hard; however, you have to keep your eyes on the prize. And no, you cannot switch up to decaffeinated coffee since, just like regular coffee, decaf contains acids that stir up your cortisol, blood sugar and your cholesterol levels. It also raises your blood pressure and affects your nervous system activity.

Basically, start cutting back on caffeine on the very first day you start the hormone reset diet (on meatless).

*Day 1-3:* say bye-bye to the last cup of coffee and drop your caffeine intake to half.

*Day 3-5:* have a mug of black tea but no more than 2 cups.

*Day 6- 8:* move to either white or green tea but not more than 2 cups on days 6 and 8. Have just 1 cup on day 8.

*Day 10:* Try to drink herbal tea.

## Caffeine Free Rules

In addition to the other rules, follow the following to reset cortisol.

**#1.** Avoid all forms of caffeine, and this includes coffee, tea (black, white, green), energy drinks and soda. Alternatives for caffeine include herbal teas, mushroom teas, hot water with cardamom/lemon and cayenne etc.

**#2.** Stick to net carbs that are between 20 grams and 49 grams a day. Net cargs is the total grams in carbs less the fiber in grams. Net carbs are the ones that raise your blood sugar and cause you to store fat.

**#3.** Keep eating a pound of veggies a day together with healthy plant-based proteins and fats and a small serving of fruits with a low glycemic index.

# Grain-Free: For Resetting Thyroid

Most of the grains out there have a high glycemic index, which means that 1- 2 hours after eating them your blood sugar spikes. As you know by now, foods that cause surges to blood sugar are not great since they lead to constant cravings and most definitely weight gain. Another downside to grains is that they contain fewer nutrients compared to animals and plants.

But grains do much more than making it difficult to lose weight; they affect the hormone thyroid.

## Thyroid And Weight

The protein gluten (found in most grains) resembles that of the thyroid tissue. When the gluten crosses the gut barrier, your immune system prepares for offense and the thyroid tissue just gets caught up in the attack.

When this happens, this means that your body will be unable to produce enough of the thyroid hormone, which leads to hypothyroidism. Thyroid hormones help in regulating your metabolism; therefore, hypothyroidism means that your metabolism will slow down, which will make it difficult to lose weight.

## Grain-Free Rules

Make sure you stock your pantry with enough foods that don't contain and follow the following rules in addition to the others:

**#1.** Cut back on all grains and flour- even gluten-free. These include:

- Cereal, bread, and any other food made with grains- even the gluten-free

- Barley, oat, rye, wheat, corn, millet, rice, spelt and any other type of grain flour/ingredients and by-products made from those grains

- Processed foods that contain wheat, grains, gluten derivatives or thickeners; these include foods such as hot dogs, mustard, luncheon meats, pickles, salad dressings, dried soup mixes, ice cream, processed cheese, pickles, beer, spices, cream sauces, non-dairy creamers and more. Just make sure you study labels.

- Gluten-free carbs. Refined carbs, gluten or not, mess up with the insulin hormone, which can block your body's ability to burn fat. So don't switch up to gluten-free options.

- Artificial flavors and seasonings. Read labels and avoid foods with ingredients such as flavoring and natural flavoring, seasoning, hydrolyzed vegetable protein, modified food starch, and maltodextrin, which all could be sourced from wheat and have gluten.

**#2:** Eat a pound of high fiber veggies each day. Women should ideally have 3 to 4 cups of leafy greens such as kale, lettuce and broccoli.

**#3.** Restrict your net carbohydrates. Ideally, aim for 20 to 49 net carbs a day to lose weight and 50 to 99 carbs to maintain your weight. But all these could depend on your current metabolism and genetics.

**#4.** Consume clean proteins. These include organic poultry, eggs and seafood about 8 to 12 ounces a day which is 80 to 110 grams. If beans don't make you feel bloated, then you can eat 1½ cup a day.

**#5.** Have only low-glycemic fruits like berries, avocados, olives and coconut. Stay away from dried fruits and fruit juices.

## Alternatives For Grains

Kelp noodles in place of pasta and noodles

Instead of buns and bread, use romaine lettuce

Coconut flour in place of wheat/ grain flour

Coconut wraps in place of carb-filled tortillas- they are a delicious alternative and are made with coconut meat and water.

If you are craving a crunchy and salty experience, try roasted seaweed in place of chips and crackers. Seaweed is an excellent source of iodine and is readily available in health food stores and supermarkets.

You can also have flaxseed and dehydrated veggie crackers.

# Dairy-Free: For Resetting Growth Hormone

Our love for dairy begins at birth with a mother's breast milk known as the healthiest food for her baby. But our bodies are designed for human breast milk, but as for cow's milk? The debate is still on. There is a protein in milk known as casein that is known to cause inflammation in our bodies and can lead to weight gain.

If you feel bloated and you keep belching or burping after having milk, then this might be it. Your immune system identifies this protein as a harmful agent (remember the case with gluten's mistaken identity) hence fires off antibodies to fight the protein. This process triggers tons of body chemicals throughout the body and can actually make it difficult to lose weight.

Let us look at the effect dairy has on the growth hormone and how that hinders weight loss.

## Growth Hormone, Dairy And Weight Loss

When it comes to the growth hormone, the problem is with the synthetic growth hormone known as 'bovine somatotropin,' which has been in the market from 1994 and is injected to approximately a third of the US 9 million dairy cows. It is injected to fatten and increase a cow's milk production by 10 to 15% if injected once every two weeks.

Well, you don't have to be a scientist to figure out that if growth hormone fattens cows, then the same effect can be experienced by your body if you consume their products. In other words, you consume a significant amount of synthetic growth hormone, which affects your hormones and leads to the storage of fat.

## Dairy-Free Rules

By now, you have already experienced the beauty of cutting back the explained conventional foods for the various hormone resets. It's now time to experience even more benefits by cutting back on dairy. Hang in there, you have six more days until you start adding back foods gradually as you track your response to the foods.

As you cut back on dairy, make room for alkaline-forming foods that are packed with iron, fiber and minerals. In addition to the other rules from the previous resets, follow the following rules:

**#1.** Avoid all of the following: yogurt, butter, milk, cheese, and kefir.

**#2.** Ensure you are getting enough protein in the form of all the allowed proteins as per the rules.

**#3.** Have a lot of fresh veggies and fiber to keep you full.

**#4.** Substitute the usual butter with pastured ghee- it has the milk solids removed and is totally casein free.

**#5.** Get foods and products that are labeled 'vegan' in supermarkets as it means they don't contain any dairy. Some include non-dairy cheeses and 'vegannaise.' Make sure though you check the labels to make sure they don't contain any casein.

**#6.** Make yourself some creamy nondairy soups that can last for up to 3 days.

### *Milk alternatives that you can consume*

Almond milk which is excellent with gluten-free cookies and smoothies- make sure it is unsweetened

Coconut milk that is made from coconuts- has a fantastic taste and can be drunk as it is, use it for cooking or in smoothies

Hemp milk- most digestible if you have gut problems

Coconut kefir- dairy-free and gluten-free and a great source of fermented food

## Toxin Free: For Resetting Testosterone

The sad truth is, environmental exposure is way too prevalent in this day and age. A lot of the foods that you consume are probably GM (Genetically Modified) and are sprayed with fertilizers and pesticides. As careful as you might be to avoid GM at home, you might go out and order steak from a cow injected with synthetic hormones.

It's not just toxicity in the foods we consume but also the cosmetics we use, the water we drink and the household cleaning products used. Not only does toxicity increase the probability of suffering from certain diseases but also it prevents your body from being able to lose weight. This reset is all about detoxification for not only resetting your testosterone but also your body and so many more hormones in your system.

### Testosterone And Weight

Testosterone is usually considered as a male hormone, but it is also present in females. It helps strengthen your muscles and bones, keeps your libido in check and enables you to burn fat.

But lifestyle factors and toxicity can lead to a significant reduction of this hormone, which can cause obesity. Going toxin-free will, however, flip this switch towards repair, healing and fat loss.

## The Science Behind Toxin-Free

As the last reset, toxin-free is a general reset that works on the whole body by ridding it of toxins. Toxins disrupt the molecular structure of your body. Eventually, toxins make you numb to hormones such as all the ones we are trying to reset in this book leading to all the adverse effects you have learned, from increased inflammation, stroke, and lowered immunity to vulnerability to autoimmune disorders.

Toxin-free focuses on getting rid of synthetic chemicals and lowering exposure to the same. It also helps your body to get rid of toxin build-up to help you live your life with clarity and lightness.

## Toxin-Free Rules

Together with the other rules, make your detox more intense by following the below rules:

**#1.** Be cautious of the products you put on your skin and mucosal membrane such as your mouth. Ensure the product that the products you use do not contain toxins. Ensure you use products such as organic deodorant and toothpaste, natural conditioner and shampoos, biodynamic lotions, and soaps.

**#2.** Increase your intake of alkaline-forming foods. An effortless way to do this is by having a cup of hot lemon water in the morning and a green shake for breakfast. You should have 2 -3 servings of greens a day.

**#3.** Continue with a pound or more of veggies daily. Cruciferous vegetables and alliums are especially great for liver detoxification so make sure you have some Brussel sprouts, cabbage, broccoli, onions and scallions.

**#4.** Your daily fiber consumption should be between 35 to 45 grams a day. You can have even higher amounts if you have no bloating or gas after. Fiber is excellent at binding metabolic blockers.

**#5.** Add spices and seeds to your cooking to improve liver detoxification. These include dill and caraway seeds, turmeric, thyme, rosemary, oregano and thyme.

**#6.** Ensure the containers you store your food in are safe by making sure they are stainless steel or glass; avoid plastic containers.

**#7.** Get out! According to the Environmental Protection Agency, the air inside our homes is about five times more polluted than the air outside. During this reset, spend more time outside, open all your windows at your home, run a HEPA filter, and replace all toxic home cleaning agents. A brisk walk outside for a couple of minutes or replacing a few products will do just fine.

You can use safer ingredients for cleaning, such as white vinegar, herbs, olive oil, borax and lemon juice.

# Chapter 3: Reentry And Sustenance

Now that you have successfully reset your hormones, you now need to preserve your acquired habits. This means that you have to be careful with reentry. As close as the end may seem, introducing foods that interfered with some of your hormones before the body is ready is not recommended.

Reentry starts from day 22 and lasts for as long as you will require gathering up data and integrating information (you might find that you need more time as most people usually add back about 3 foods only between days 22 and 30).

During reentry ensure you add back one food at a time to see how exactly your body responds. This will help you be more aware of your body and the foods that are not great for you that you need to avoid altogether.

## Developing A Personal Food Code

This should be your first step in reentry. A personal food code states (in writing) your personal commitment when it comes to nourishment and food. Writing down will help you track down even the minutest detail and adjustments that your body makes in response to the food you eat. The reentry phase gives you the opportunity to edit your personal food code to meet your external and internal demands.

When drafting it, ensure you put into consideration the kind of relationship to health and food that you mostly desire. The idea here is to come up with boundaries regarding food that you can live by. It can be long or short; whatever works for you.

Once you have it drafted, revisit it and revise it as much as you need to make sure its practical and actually works for you.

## Reentry: The Three-Day Challenge

With reentry or re-introduction, you will be adding back a food at a time and then observing your body's response for 3 days. Follow the following reentry steps for a smooth experience:

**#1.** Have a journal and draft your personal food code in it.

**#2.** Pick your challenge food- the one you craved the most or had the hardest time giving up- sometimes that is the food that you are most reactive to.

**#3.** Eat the selected food in one meal at the beginning of day 22. Have the food again on day 23 and 24; basically, the same food and only just once a day.

**#4.** Try, tweak and triumph. Keep an eye on your body's response for those 3 days, including food-mood connection, what happens to your pulse, gut (gurgling, bloating, bowel movements, gas) and body (pains, discomfort and aches). You can use measurements and techniques such as blood sugar, pulse, food-mood journaling and measuring weight.

**#5.** Once you have a clear record of your reactions over 3 days, pick your next challenge food for test during the next 3 days.

**#6.** If you feel like you need to take the reintroduction slower than this then that is okay. But don't do it faster. People are different and you might find that you may need to be on this diet longer to reap benefits such as improved blood sugar and weight loss.

**#7.** You don't have to reintroduce all the foods you eliminated. For example, you might choose to not introduce back sugar, grains and dairy. In accordance to this, your length of reentry will depend on the foods you chose to add back.

# Sustenance

This is all about sustaining your progress and keeping your reset hormones in check. Briefly, the gateway to sustaining weight for life is by keeping your insulin balanced. You might not have lost as much weight as you had planned but if you do a hormone reset each quarter (after every 3 months), you will achieve your weight loss goals.

## The Three Sustenance Rules

**#1.** Stay away from refined carbs. As you already know, foods with low glycemic index leads to lesser release of insulin and inflammation, which is great for achieving a lean body. On the contrary, refined carbs such as sugar, bread, pizza, pasta, starches etc., trigger the release of insulin, the fat-storing hormone.

**#2.** Eat adequate protein. This is so important because protein keeps you fuller for longer, and avoids instances of unnecessary snacking.

**#3.** Keep an eye on triglycerides and net carbs. Triglycerides are the fats that your liver makes constantly as you overindulge in carbs and further low fiber sources of fructose. These fats are notorious in clogging your arteries that is why you should stick to nutrient dense veggies, clean proteins and healthy fats.

## Further Strategies To Help With Sustenance

*Have breakfast regularly-* a healthy breakfast will help keep you from snacking throughout the day.

### *Exercise consistently*

**Self-monitoring-** keeping track of your progress e.g. how food affects you, your weight loss/gain over time to have some sort of control when it comes to your weight.

**Stick to a consistent eating pattern-** this is across weekends, weekdays and even holidays.

# Chapter 4: Hormone Reset Diet Recipes

## Breakfast Recipes

### Hazelnut Chocolate Shake

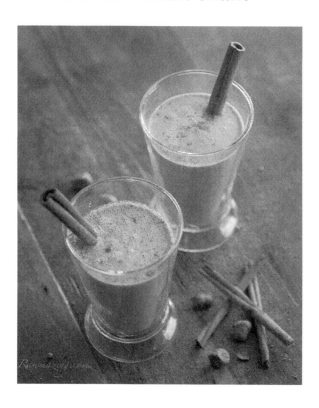

# Hormone Reset Diet Meal Plan

*Serves 1*

*Ingredients*

1 tablespoon pure cacao powder

1-inch piece of fresh ginger, peeled and chopped

1 tablespoon turmeric

1 tablespoon cashew butter

1 cup raw kale

1 cup unsweetened hazelnut milk

1 tablespoon raw cacao nibs

2 tablespoons chia seeds, soaked (optional)

2 scoops organic protein powder

*Directions*

Toss all ingredients into a high-powered blender and blend until smooth.

Pour into a tall glass/mason jar and drink up.

*Garnish with cinnamon sticks if desired.

## Breakfast Liver Tonic

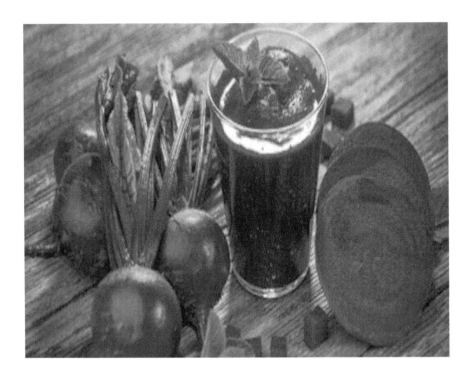

*Serves 3 to 4*

*Ingredients*

Juice of one red grapefruit

2-inch piece of fresh ginger, peeled and chopped

2 cinnamon sticks

2 medium beets, peeled and sliced

2-inch piece of fresh turmeric, peeled and chopped

½ cup fresh mint leaves

6 cups filtered water

8 to 10 leaves of dandelion greens

1 cup broccoli sprouts

4 or 5 large leaves of red chard

## Directions

Add beets, cinnamon sticks and water to a large pot and place over high heat. Once it boils, cook for about 20 to 30 minutes until the beets are tender.

Sieve the beets and discard the cinnamon sticks and water. In a high-powered blender, blend the beets, turmeric, chard, mint, ginger, broccoli sprouts, dandelion greens and grapefruit juice then add this mixture to the pot.

Allow the tonic to heat over low heat for about 1 to 2 hours.

Serve cold or warm.

# Chocolate Cherry Smoothie

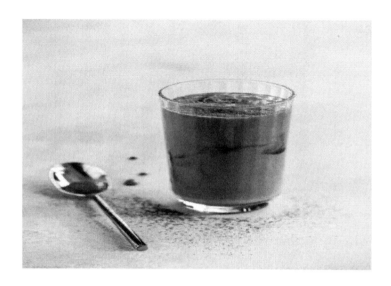

*Serves 2*

*Ingredients*

½ teaspoon cinnamon powder

1 avocado

1 teaspoon vanilla extract

A handful of hazelnuts, soaked overnight

1 tablespoon coconut butter

A handful of dry cherries, pre-soak in water for about 10 minutes

1 teaspoon lemon or lime juice

A handful of pumpkin seeds

2 tablespoons raw unsweetened cacao

### *Directions*

Add all ingredients into blender and run it until smooth.

Pour into a glass and enjoy.

## Sweet Potato Waffle Sandwich

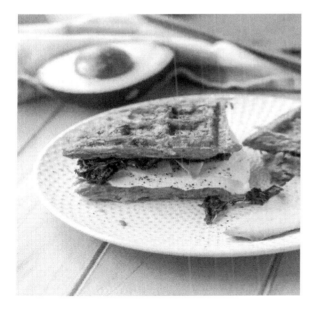

*Serves 2*

*Ingredients*

1/2 medium avocado, sliced

1 medium sweet potato, grated

1/8 teaspoon garlic salt

2 large eggs- divided

1 teaspoon oil, plus more for waffle iron and frying pan

1/8 teaspoon paprika

1 cup kale, chopped

1/4 teaspoon cumin

Salt and pepper- to taste

*Directions*

Heat the waffle iron and coat with oil. Set aside.

Whisk the eggs in a mixing bowl and add in the grated sweet potato (around a heaping cup), 1 teaspoon of oil and seasonings.

Combine thoroughly and once the waffle iron is heated, pack the sweet potato hash in. Ensure you cover all the quadrants then press the iron down gently. Let the waffle cook for approximately 4 to 5 minutes until golden lightly.

As the waffle cooks, fry the kale with oil over medium heat until a bit crispy, this should take about 3 to 4 minutes. Scramble or fry the egg in the same pan; you can remove or keep the kale as desired.

Once the waffle cooks, use a butter knife to remove gently and onto a plate. Add the fried egg, kale and avocado slices to the waffle in layers. Season with some pepper and salt as desired and enjoy.

### Recipe notes

Try to squeeze out the water from the sweet potato before mixing in the rest of the ingredients to make the waffle firmer.

Also ensure you grease the waffle iron well to prevent burning.

## Sweet Potato Pancakes

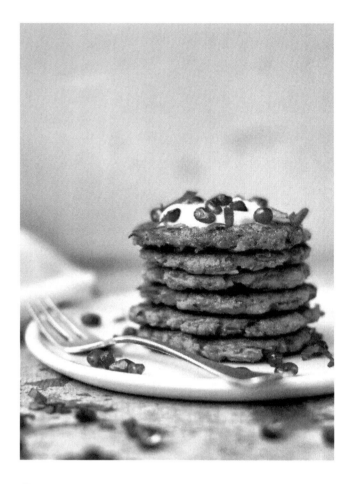

*Serves 10*

*Ingredients*

1/2 teaspoon pepper

1/4 cup chickpea flour

1/4 teaspoon paprika

1/4 teaspoon cayenne pepper

1/2 small yellow onion- shredded

1 tablespoon apple cider vinegar

1/2 teaspoon sea salt

1/2 teaspoon cumin

1 1/2 cups sweet potato, shredded

2 tablespoons water

1 tablespoon olive oil

Coconut oil for cooking

## *Directions*

Add the onion and sweet potato into a large bowl and add in the oil, water, chickpea flour, spices and vinegar. Use your hands or a wooden spoon to mix well ensuring no flour streaks can be seen; set aside.

Place a large flat bottomed pan over medium heat to warm then add a bit of coconut oil (or oil of choice). Use your hands to form a ball from the sweet potato mixture and flatten between your hands to achieve about 2-cm thickness.

Put onto the hot pan and cook for a minute until golden, flip and cook the other side for a minute. You can cook 3 or 4 at a time but check not to crowd the pan. Repeat this with all the batter.

You can add the cooked pancakes in a warm oven to keep warm.

Serve while hot with your desired toppings

Enjoy!

### *Recipe notes*

The mixture might be extra wet depending on how dense your sweet potato is- don't worry they it will come together once you fry them.

You can also use sweet or smoked paprika, which will be as amazing.

# Chickpea Scramble

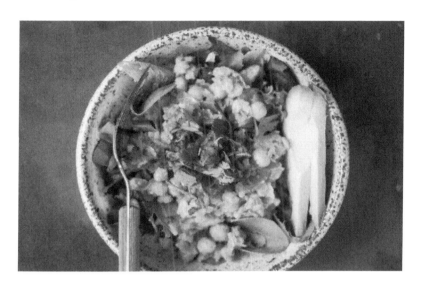

*Serves 2*

*Ingredients*

Chickpea Scramble:

Drizzle of extra virgin olive oil

2 cloves garlic, minced

½ teaspoon salt

1 15 ounces can of chickpeas

½ teaspoon pepper

¼ white onion, diced

½ teaspoon turmeric

### *Breakfast Bowl:*

Handful of Cilantro, minced

Avocado

Mixed Greens

Handful of Parsley, minced

### *Directions*

### *Chickpea Scramble:*

Pour out the chickpeas into a bowl, add some water and mash slightly using a fork. Add in the pepper, salt and turmeric and mix well until nicely combined.

Dice the onion and mince the garlic. Place a pan over medium flame to heat then add some olive oil. Add the onions and cook until they are soft.

Add in the garlic and continue frying for about a minute until the garlic is fragrant but make sure the garlic does not brown.

Once the garlic and onions are done, add in mashed chickpeas and cook for about 5 minutes.

### *For the breakfast bowls:*

To assemble the bowls, add mixed greens at the bottom of the bowls and top with the chickpea scramble. Top with some minced parsley and cilantro. Serve with some avocado slices.

Enjoy!

## Berry Coconut Breakfast Bowl

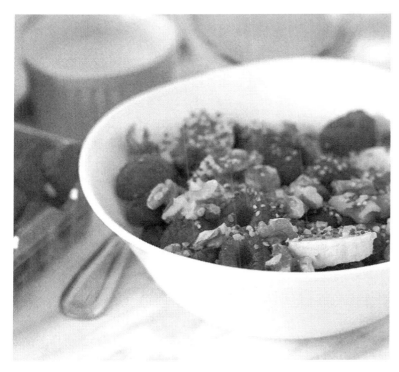

*Serves 1*

*Ingredients*

2 teaspoons hemp hearts (optional)

2 tablespoons chopped walnuts

1 cup mixed berries, washed

2 teaspoons chia seeds

¼ cup coconut milk

1 sliced banana- omit if you've reached fruitless

*Directions*

Add the chopped walnuts, berries and sliced banana to a bowl. Sprinkle some hemp (if using) and chia seeds on top.

Pour in the coconut milk, mix and enjoy.

# Cauliflower Tortillas

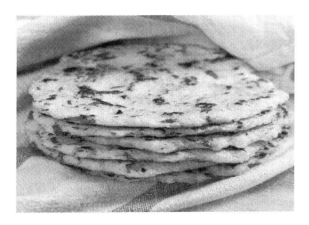

## *Yield 6 tortillas*

## *Ingredients*

Salt and pepper, to taste

1/2 lime, juiced and zested

1/4 cup chopped fresh cilantro

¾ large head cauliflower (or two cups riced)

2 large eggs (substitute flax eggs for vegan)

## *Directions*

Preheat your oven to 375 degrees F and use parchment paper to line a baking sheet. Trim your cauliflower and chop into

53

small and uniform pieces then put into a food processor in batches to pulse.

Once you get a couscous like consistency, stop; you should get about 2 cups packed of finely riced cauliflower. Add the cauliflower to a microwave safe bowl and cook for 2 minutes, stir then cook for 2 more minutes in the microwave- a steamer will work just as well.

Put the cauliflower onto a thin dishtowel or a fine cheesecloth and squeeze out as much liquid as you can; watch out so that you don't burn yourself or use dishwashing gloves to do this.

Whisk eggs in a medium bowl and add in cilantro, cauliflower, pepper, salt and lime. Mix well to combine then using your hands, create 6 small 'tortillas' on parchment paper.

Bake in oven for 10 minutes, carefully flip then cook again for about 5 to 7 more minutes or until set completely. Put onto a wire rack to cool a bit.

Place a medium sized skillet over medium heat and add baked tortillas to the pan. Press down slightly and brown for about 1 to 2 minutes on both sides. Do this with all the tortillas.

### *Recipe Notes*

You can eat them alone or make some quesadillas with them. You can also add some taco filling and fold like a taco and enjoy.

You can use already riced cauliflower instead of processing a cauliflower head.

Leftovers freeze quite well.

# Lunch Recipes

## Zucchini Noodles With Arugula Pesto

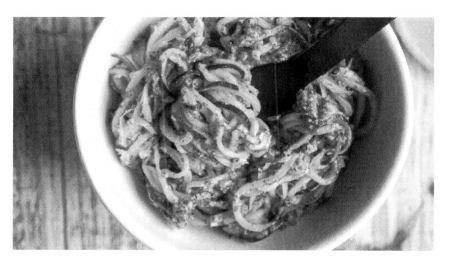

*Serves 4 to 6*

*Ingredients*

4 cups fresh arugula

⅓ cup olive oil

2 tablespoons full-fat, unsweetened coconut milk

2 large zucchini- or 4 or 5 small zucchini

1 or 2 cloves fresh garlic- depending on taste

Zest of one lemon

½ teaspoon black pepper

Juice of one lemon

3 tablespoons nutritional yeast

1 teaspoon garlic salt

1 tablespoon coconut oil

**Directions**

Use a julienne peeler to peel the zucchini into long slices lengthwise- they are supposed to look like spaghetti noodles. Set aside.

Blend the lemon juice, pepper, garlic salt and coconut milk in a food processor and once smooth, add in the garlic cloves, arugula, olive oil, lemon zest, nutritional yeast and blend again until creamy.

Add coconut oil in a large skillet and heat over medium high heat. Add in your zucchini noodles and cook in batches-depending on the size of your skillet. Fry until the zucchini noodles just brighten; this should take about 4 to 6 minutes.

Remove the zucchini from the heat and serve with prepared pesto.

Enjoy!

## Beet And Carrot Salad

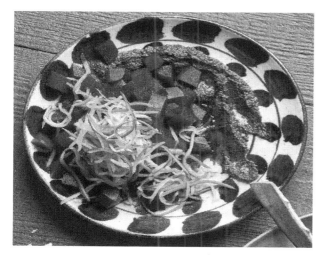

***Serves 4 to 6***

***Ingredients***

*For the Salad*

2 cups shredded carrots

¼ cup chopped scallions

¼ cup chopped fresh flat-leaf parsley

2 cups peeled, shredded raw beets

1 cup chopped raw walnuts

*For the Dressing*

1 teaspoon ground cumin

½ cup extra-virgin olive oil

Zest of one orange

¼ cup freshly squeezed orange juice

1 teaspoon salt

2 tablespoons apple cider vinegar

## *Directions*

Combine all the salad ingredients in a large bowl to make the salad.

To make the dressing, add all dressing ingredients to a jar, seal with lid and shake well to combine.

Add dressing to salad and toss to coat. Serve chilled at room temperature.

This salad can keep in the fridge well for up to 4 days.

## Paleo Grilled Sweet Potatoes

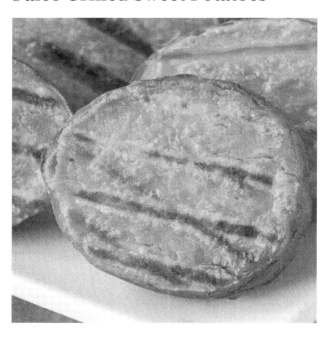

*Serves 4*

*Ingredients*

1 tablespoon stevia

1 tablespoon sea salt

3- 4 sweet potatoes cut into discs

1 tablespoon coconut oil

1 teaspoon smoked paprika optional

1 teaspoon red pepper flakes optional

*Directions*

Preheat your grill or barbeque to medium and coat it well with cooking spray or brush generously with coconut oil.

Put the sweet potato and coconut oil into a large mixing bowl and mix. Add in sweetener, smoked paprika, sea salt and red pepper flakes and combine to coat the sweet potatoes well.

Layer the discs on the grill and cook for about 12 to 15 minutes, flipping once soft and charred on one side.

Serve the sweet potatoes with some sautéed vegetables for a complete meal.

## *Recipe notes*

Do not exceed 2 or 3 tablespoons with the oil as the sweet potatoes will get stuck on the grill and become too soft. The cooking time also depends on the temperature and power of the grill.

Left overs can keep in the fridge in a sealed container for up to 3 days.

## **Sweet Potato Noodles With Cashew Sauce**

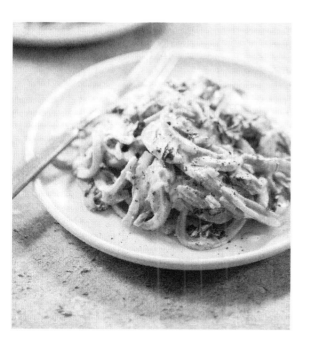

*Serves 4 to 6*

*Ingredients*

1/2 teaspoon salt

3/4 cup water

1 tablespoon oil

4 large sweet potatoes, spiralized

1 clove garlic

A handful of basil leaves or any other herbs

2 cups baby spinach

1 cup cashews

Olive oil for drizzling

Salt and pepper to taste

*Directions*

Add the cashews to a bowl of water and cover for about 2 hours. Drain and then rinse with water thoroughly.

Put the cashews into a food processor or blender and add garlic, salt and ¾ cup of water; blend until very smooth.

Add oil to a large skillet and heat over medium-high heat. Add in the sweet potatoes and cook as you toss with tongs until crispy and tender. Remove from the heat and add in the spinach- it will wilt pretty quickly.

Toss in half of the herbs and half of the sauce in the pan and combine well. If the mixture is too sticky, add some water. Season with some pepper and salt generously and drizzle with olive oil. Top with the rest of the fresh herbs. Enjoy!

### *Recipe Notes*

The recipe makes sauce enough for at least 6 to 8 servings if not more (just enough for this recipe wouldn't be enough to go through the blender). Don't worry, you will be able to make use of the extra sauce, as it is super versatile.

The size of the sweet potatoes affects greatly the number of servings for this recipe.

The recipe also gives tons of flavor so feel free to add whatever flavors or herbs you want to give the sauce more of a punch. Roasted garlic and caramelized onions maybe?

## Sweet & Tangy Bean Salad

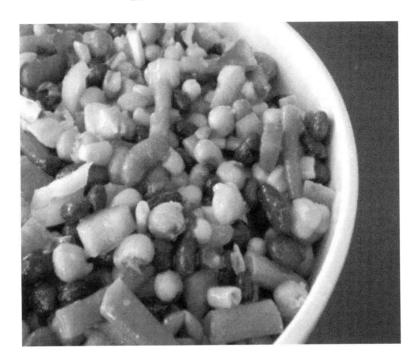

*Serves 8*

*Ingredients*

¼ cup of chopped green pepper

2 cans of yellow wax beans, drained

½ cup of white vinegar

½ cup of canola or olive oil

¼ cup of chopped white or red onion

1 can of chickpeas, drained

1 can of red kidney beans, drained/rinsed

½ cup of stevia

Salt and pepper to taste

2 cans of cut green beans, drained

## *Directions*

Drain and thoroughly rinse the beans and add them to a bowl. Add in the stevia, oil and vinegar. Add in chopped onions and green pepper and stir again.

Add pepper and salt to taste then combine the ingredients well.

Place in the fridge for 8 hours before you serve.

To make this dish perfectly, consider remixing it every 1 to 2 hours for enhanced flavors.

## Cauliflower Mushroom Risotto

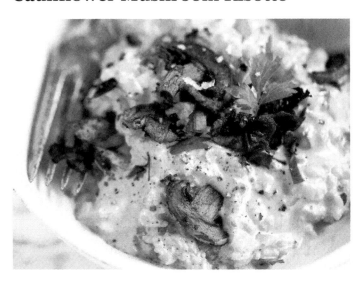

*Serves 4*

*Ingredients*

*Cauli Rice:*

1 tablespoon olive oil

8 cups cauliflower rice

*Cheese Sauce:*

1 1/2 teaspoons sea salt

1/2 teaspoon paprika

3/4 cup raw cashews

1 cup full fat coconut milk- shake can before using

1/4 cup nutritional yeast

2 cloves garlic

*Mushrooms:*

2 tablespoons fresh minced parsley

1 teaspoon olive oil

8 white mushrooms sliced

Salt and pepper to taste

Truffle oil to taste

*Toppings:*

Freshly ground pepper

Lemon wedges

Sea salt flakes

¼ cup chopped fresh basil or parsley

## *Directions*

Sauté cauliflower rice in a large fry pan with a tablespoon of olive oil for 3-4 minutes over medium heat on the stove. Once soft (but not mushy) remove from the stove.

Add all the cheese sauce ingredients to a high-powered blender and blend on high for a couple of minutes until combined and smooth.

Add all the mushroom ingredients onto a baking tray lined with parchment paper and toss to combine well. Toast in a toaster oven for a few minutes until a bit crispy and cooked. You can just bake in the oven as well.

Once cooked, pour the cheese sauce all over the cauliflower rice and top with the mushrooms and toppings.

Enjoy!

# Power Bowl

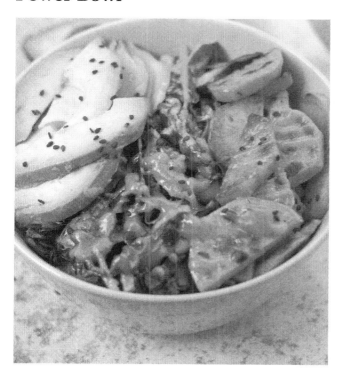

*Serves 1*

*Ingredients*

¾ teaspoon + 1 ½ teaspoons coconut oil- divided

1 teaspoon coconut oil

1 soft boiled egg

1 cup sliced sweet potatoes

2 cups sliced cabbage

1/2 sliced Hass avocado

*Tangy Cashew Dressing*

½ teaspoon apple cider vinegar

2 teaspoons olive oil

2 teaspoons cashew butter

*Garnish*

Black sesame seeds

## Directions

Melt the ¾ teaspoon of coconut oil in a medium pan over medium to high heat and add in the sliced cabbage. Toss as you cook for 5 to 8 minutes or until the cabbage wilts slightly. Once ready, remove from the heat and set aside.

In a different pot, add 2 cups of water and bring to a boil. Add the remaining coconut oil in the pan you fried the cabbage, heat it up and then add the sliced sweet potatoes making sure you distribute them evenly.

Cook for about 5 minutes then flip the potatoes and cook for 5 more minutes; remove from heat. Add the egg to boiling water and allow to sit for about 5 minutes. Remove from the boiled water and dunk the egg in an ice bath.

Assemble your power bowl; add cooked cabbage and sweet potatoes plus half sliced avocado.

For the cashew dressing, combine the cashew butter, olive oil and apple cider vinegar and combine well.

Drizzle the dressing on top of your bowl and peel the cooled egg gently and place on top.

Garnish with some black sesame seeds and enjoy!

## Sweet Potato & Carrot Salad

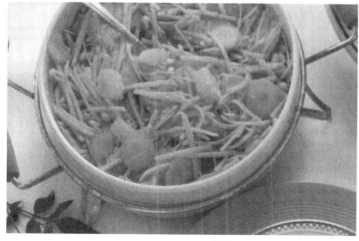

*Serves 2*

*Ingredients*

½ grapefruit (juice and pulp)- omit if you've reached fruitless

1 large sweet potato

1 orange (juice and pulp)- omit if you've reached fruitless

2 tablespoons of olive oil

1/3 cup of pine nuts

½ lemon (juice and a little zest)

2 large carrots

*Directions*

Peel the sweet potato and carrot (leave the peel if they are organic but scrub well to clean). Use a mandolin or spiralizer to make small juliennes of sweet potato or spaghetti type swirls.

Thinly slice your carrots using your mandolin then add to the salad bowl. Juice the orange and grapefruit (optional) and pull out the pulp for each fruit. Juice and zest the lemon too and pour this over the sweet potato and carrot mixture.

Season with salt and drizzle with olive oil and combine well.

Put the salad in the fridge and let it marinade for about an hour. Turn over every 20 minutes or so until ready to serve.

Garnish with the pine nuts.

Serve and enjoy!

# Dinner Recipes

## Lemon Zoodles

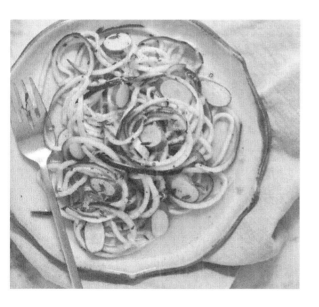

***Serves 4***

***Ingredients***

1 tablespoon chopped fresh thyme

½ teaspoon garlic powder

½ teaspoon Dijon mustard

3 medium zucchini, cut into noodles

Salt and freshly ground black pepper

1 lemon, zested and juiced

1 bunch radishes, thinly sliced

⅓ cup olive oil

***Directions***

Add lemon zest, mustard, lemon juice and garlic powder to a small bowl and whisk to combine.

Add in the olive oil bit by bit as you whisk to combine; season with some pepper and salt.

Toss the radishes with the zucchini in a large bowl and add in the dressing. Toss to coat the veggies well.

Serve right away garnished with some fresh thyme.

## Cauliflower Fried Rice

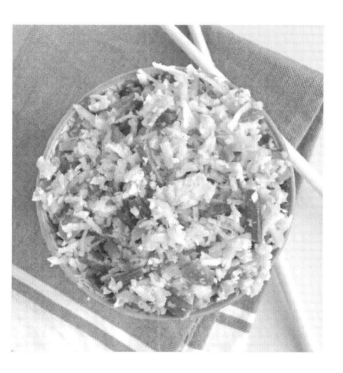

*Serves 4*

*Ingredients*

½ teaspoon garlic powder

Salt to taste

1 tablespoon coconut oil

¼ cup + 1 tablespoon Coconut Aminos

½ cup chopped carrots

2 eggs

1 cup chopped green beans

½ teaspoon pepper

1 head of cauliflower chopped (about 4 –5 cups)

¼ cup chopped onions

### *Directions*

Heat a large skillet over medium high heat and add a tablespoon of coconut oil to heat up. Add in the chopped onions and allow to cook for 2 minutes as you stir occasionally. Toss in the cauliflower and cook until it starts to get tender; about 5 minutes.

Place the chopped green beans in a microwavable bowl together with a splash of water. Microwave for 2 minutes on high; this will cook them perfectly so as to move things along quicker.

Pour out water, green beans and carrots to the mixture with cauliflower and stir to combine. Make a deep well in the middle of the pan by pushing the mixture to the sides.

Mix the eggs, a few grinds of pepper and a pinch of salt in a small bowl. Pour this mixture into the well of the pan and stir but make sure not to combine with the cauliflower mixture. When the eggs are scrambled, stir together with the cauliflower mixture.

Add in the garlic, coconut aminos and pepper. Season to taste with salt if need be. Stir to combine, taste the seasonings and adjust the tastes as desired.

Green Detox Soup

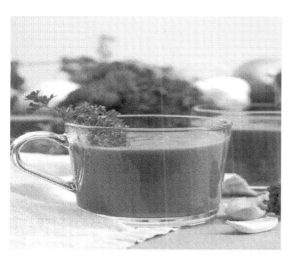

***Serves 6***

***Ingredients***

3 zucchinis, sliced

2 tablespoons of coconut oil

2 sprigs of fresh thyme- removed from stem

3 tablespoons of fresh mint

3 cloves of garlic, minced

1 ½ cups of frozen peas

2 cups of fine green beans, chopped

Salt and pepper- to taste

5 cups of vegetable stock

1 white onion, finely diced

1 ½ cups of broccoli florets

***Directions***

Add coconut oil to a large pot and heat. Toss in the garlic and onion and fry the onions until soft; about 8 minutes.

Toss in the green beans, peas, broccoli and zucchini and cook for a couple of minutes. Now add in thyme, veggie stock and mint to the pot. Let it boil then simmer for 30 minutes.

Pour the vegetables into a blender or use a stick blender and blend until you achieve desired consistency.

Season with salt and pepper and enjoy while hot.

## Caprese

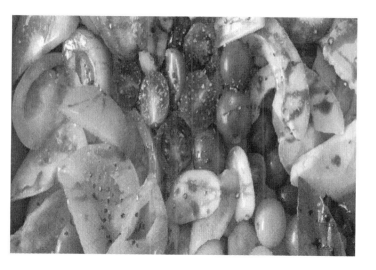

### *Ingredients*

*Salad*

Tomatoes

Avocados

Olives

Hearts of palm

Cucumbers

*Dressing*

Kosher salt and freshly ground black pepper to taste

¼ cup fresh mint- chopped

1 cup basil- chopped

1 tablespoon high quality balsamic vinegar

¼ cup extra virgin olive oil

### **Directions**

To make the dressing, mix all the dressing ingredients thoroughly.

For the salad, cut the ingredients into nice pieces and assemble on a platter well. Take your time and make a nice pattern.

Once done, drizzle the dressing and enjoy!

# Zucchini Cauliflower Fritters

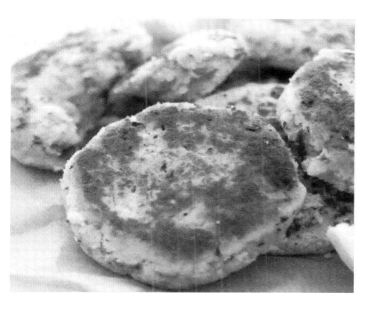

***Serves 8***

***Ingredients***

2 large eggs

2 medium zucchini

¼ teaspoon black pepper

¼ cup coconut flour

½ head cauliflower approximately 3 cups, chopped

½ teaspoon sea salt

### *Egg-Free version*

¼ cup gluten-free flour

¼ teaspoon black pepper

½ teaspoon sea salt

½ head cauliflower approximately 3 cups- chopped

2 medium zucchini

### *Directions*

Grate the zucchini in your food processor. Steam cauliflower for 5 minutes until fork tender and add the steamed cauliflower to a food processor. Process cauliflower until you have small chunks making sure not to over-process into a mash.

Using a nut milk bag or a dishtowel, squeeze out as much moisture as you can out of the grated vegetables. Transfer this to a bowl and add in flour of your choice, salt, egg if using, pepper and any other seasoning desired.

Mix well to combine and shape into small patties (it will make about 8).

Heat about 1 tablespoon of coconut oil in a large pan. Add 4 of the fritters to pan and cook for 2 to 3 minutes on each side over medium heat. Do this with the second half of the fritters.

Serve with healthy dipping sauce of your choice.

### *Recipe notes*

The fritters can are freezer friendly and can be refrigerated.

## Pan Roasted Portobello Egg

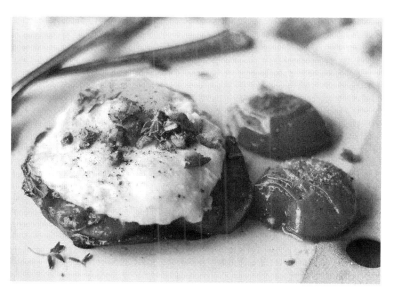

*Serves 4*

*Ingredients*

6 to 8 cloves garlic

Olive oil for cooking

4 eggs

2 portabella mushrooms

4 medium tomatoes

Salt and pepper to taste

Fresh thyme for sprinkling on top

*Directions*

Cut the mushrooms in half and oil a large frying pan with olive oil. Add mushrooms to the pan and cook for 10 minutes approximately over medium heat on the stovetop (5 minutes on each side) until soft and a bit crispy on the edges.

When the mushrooms are done cooking set them aside. Cut tomatoes in half and cook in the pan with some olive oil; enough to ensure they don't burn or stick. Cook for 5 minutes on each side (10 minutes in total) then remove and set aside once done.

Mince the garlic and fry for one minute with some olive oil until crispy and golden. Set aside.

Fry the eggs as desired then assemble your mushroom toast. Top with some crispy garlic, sea salt, fresh thyme leaves and freshly cracked pepper.

Enjoy!

## Avocado Salad

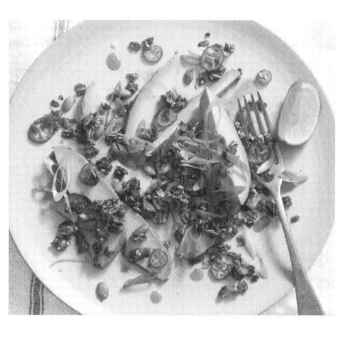

*Serves 4*

*Ingredients*

2/3 cup Spicy Sesame-Tamari Granola

½ serrano chile (very thinly sliced)

1 tablespoon chile oil

2 small avocados

½ lime

*Directions*

Slice up the avocados and arrange them nicely on a platter. Squeeze out the juice from half a lime on top and sprinkle some Serrano chile.

Drizzle chile oil and sprinkle some natural spicy sesame tamari granola.

Enjoy!

# Beet, Mushroom And Avocado Salad

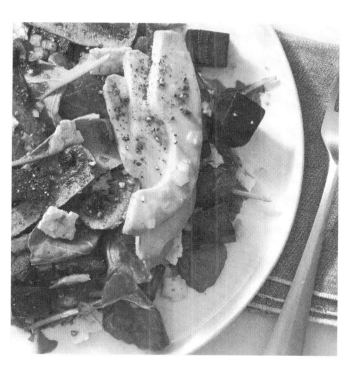

*Serves 4*

*Ingredients*

¼ cup lemon juice

2 sheets matzo- crushed into pieces (optional)

4 medium Portobello mushroom caps

8 ounces precooked beets- chopped

3 tablespoons olive oil

1 small shallot- finely chopped

2 ripe avocados- thinly sliced

5 ounces baby kale

### *Directions*

Place the mushroom caps onto a large rimmed baking sheet and spray the mushroom with nonstick cooking spray. Season with ½ teaspoon of salt and roast for 20 minutes or until tender at 450 degrees F.

Mix together lemon juice, shallot, olive oil, pepper and salt, and toss half of the mixture with the beets and baby kale. Divide between serving plates. Top with matzo (if using), Portobello and avocado, all thinly sliced.

Serve with the rest of the dressing on the side.

# Kale and Beet Salad

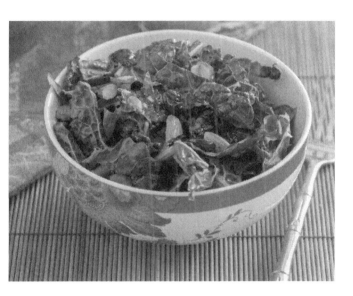

*Serves 4 to 6*

*Ingredients*

## For the dressing:

1 teaspoon thyme

2 tablespoons olive oil

Salt and pepper to taste

½ teaspoon fennel seeds

3 tablespoons red wine vinegar

**For the salad:**

1/4 red onion- thinly sliced

1/2 head of butter lettuce- chopped

1 medium beet

4 or 5 large leaves of dinosaur kale

### *Directions*

*For Dressing*

Whisk together the olive oil, fennel seeds, pepper, salt, thyme and vinegar in a small bowl and set aside.

*For Salad*

Add the beet and water in a medium pan and bring to a boil. Lower the heat and let the beets simmer until tender; about 20 to 30 minutes.

Remove the beet  from the pan and rinse with cold water. Remove the skin and chop beet into small thin pieces; set aside.

Massage kale with your fingers until the leaves turn bright green and silky in texture. Slice the massaged leaves to thin pieces.

Add the beet, onion, kale and lettuce to a large bowl and toss well. Top with the dressing.

Enjoy!

# Snack And Dessert Recipes

## Broiled Grapefruit

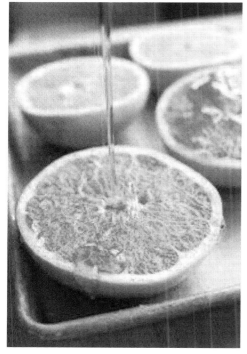

*Serves 1*

*Ingredients*

Honey

Ground ginger or ground cinnamon

Grapefruit

Optional: banana slices (strawberries are great too)

*Directions*

Set up the oven for broiling and place an oven rack at the top. Cut the grapefruit into halves and loosen the sections from the membranes using a small serrated knife or a grapefruit knife.

Add the grapefruits halves to a baking sheet or shallow baking pan and drizzle some honey. Place the banana slices on top and flip over once to coat all over with honey. Dust with some ground cinnamon or/and ginger.

Broil until bubbling and browned slightly for 4 to 6 minutes, make sure to keep a close eye to avoid burning.

Serve and enjoy while warm.

# Baked Pears With Walnuts And Honey

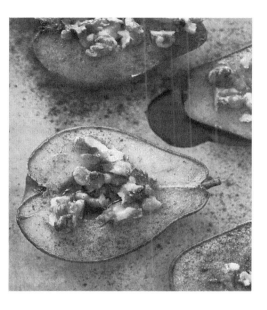

*Serves 4*

*Ingredients*

2 teaspoons of honey

2 large ripe pears

¼ cup of crushed walnuts

¼ teaspoon of ground cinnamon

Yogurt or frozen yogurt (optional)

## *Directions*

Preheat the oven to 350 degrees F and cut the pears in half. Put onto a baking sheet sheet and set the halves facing upright, and cut a sliver off the end.

Take out the seeds using a measuring spoon or baller and sprinkle some cinnamon. Sprinkle walnuts on top and drizzle half a teaspoon of honey over each half.

Bake in oven for about 30 minutes, remove and let it cool.

Enjoy!

## Avocado Ice Cream

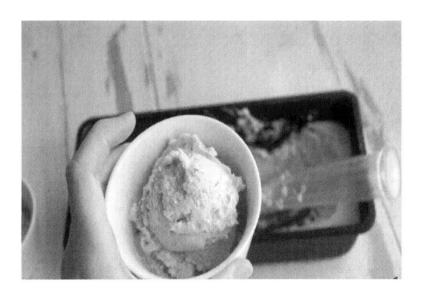

*Serves 4*

*Ingredients*

1 teaspoon lemon juice

1 ½ avocados

1 can (14 ounces) full-fat coconut milk

1/3 cup stevia

*Directions*

Place the can of coconut milk in the fridge overnight.

Chop the avocados in half and remove the pit. Spoon out the flesh and add to a food processor together with the lemon juice. Blend until perfectly smooth.

Open coconut milk can upside down such that the hard cream is on top. Scoop out the cream leaving the coconut water (save the water for a different recipe).

Whip the cream using an electrical mixer until you achieve a soft, coconut whipped cream. Add in the avocado, stevia and combine until nicely incorporated.

Put your ice cream mix in a freezer safe dish put in the freezer for at least 4 hours.

If too hard to spoon out after 4 hours, allow to sit at room temperature for a few minutes prior to digging in!

## Oil-Free Baked Curly Fries

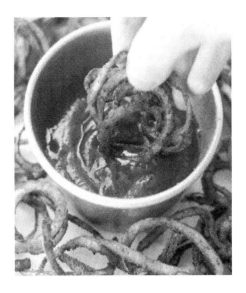

*Serves 1*

*Ingredients*

¼ teaspoon sea salt

2 teaspoons smoked paprika

¼ teaspoon onion powder

1 large russet potato

¼ teaspoon garlic powder

### *Directions*

Preheat your oven to 425 degrees F.

Combine the garlic powder, paprika, salt and onion powder in a small cup and set aside.

In a large bowl, spiralize the potato. Use kitchen scissors to cut the strips into about 6 to 8 inches lengths to prevent tangling and cooking unevenly. Sprinkle some seasonings on top of the pieces of potato and toss to coat evenly.

Spread fries out evenly on a baking sheet that is lined with parchment paper; ensure not to over crowd them. Bake for about 15 minutes at 425 degrees F.

Remove the pan from the oven and rearrange or thoroughly flip the fries such that the less cooked ones have more space.

Return back in the oven and cook for 10 minutes. After the 10 minutes, check and remove the ones that are golden brown and crispy. Put back any soft ones in the oven for 5 to 10 minutes.

Let the fries cool a bit.

Enjoy as they are or with a healthy dipping sauce of your choice.

## Almond Butter Fudge Bars

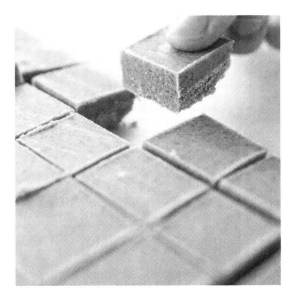

*Serves 8 to 10*

*Ingredients*

1 cup full-fat canned coconut milk

1½ cups unsweetened almond butter

2 tablespoons coconut oil

3 large pure cacao or 100 percent dark chocolate bars (4 to 6 ounces each)

1 ½ cups organic xylitol, divided

2 teaspoons pure vanilla extract- divided

**Directions**

Break the bars of chocolate into bits and put them in a double broiler or microwave to melt. Once melted, stir in the vanilla extract, coconut oil and ½ cup of xylitol.

Use parchment paper to line a shallow baking dish and pour in the chocolate mixture in an even layer at the bottom of the dish. Put in the freezer for about 30 minutes or until the chocolate is hard.

In the meantime, combine the rest of the vanilla, xylitol, almond butter and coconut milk in a large bowl; stir well to combine.

Spread this mixture all over the hardened chocolate evenly.

Cover and freeze again for about an hour. Cut into small squares and serve while cold, right from the freezer!

## Lemon cheesecake

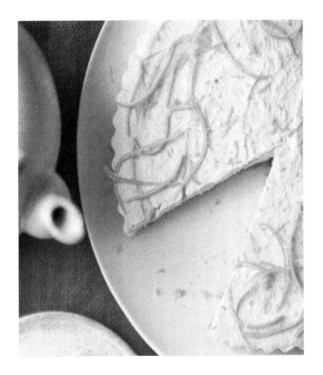

*Serves 12*

*Ingredients*

*For the base:*

30g of coconut oil, plus extra for greasing

100g of blanched almonds

100g of soft pitted dates- skip if you've reached fruitless

*For the topping:*

2 ½ tablespoons of stevia (or agave syrup)

150ml of almond milk

2 lemons, zested and juiced

300g of cashew nuts

50g of coconut oil

### Directions

Add the cashews to a large bowl and soak for 1 hour in boiling water. As they soak, add the base ingredients into your food processor and add a pinch of salt. Process the ingredients until smooth.

Grease a tart tin with coconut oil and press your mixture into the base. Add to the fridge and let it set for about 30 minutes.

Drain the water from the cashews and put in the food processor with the rest of the topping ingredients except from the ¼ zest (place this in a damp kitchen paper for serving). Process until smooth.

Spoon this mixture to the base and put in the fridge for 2 hours so that the cheesecake sets completely.

Spread the reserved lemon zest all over just before you serve.

Spoon the mixture to the base then place in the fridge for at least 2 hours to completely set

## Avocado Smoothie

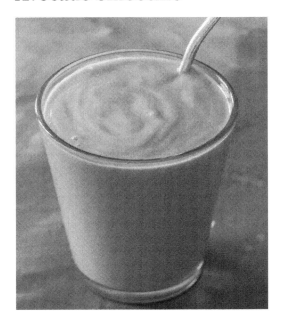

# Hormone Reset Diet Meal Plan

*Serves 2*

## Ingredients

1 tablespoon of flaxseeds

1 Avocado`

1 ½ cups of plant based milk

1 teaspoon of cinnamon

½ cup of water (for dilution) and a little ice

½ pack of frozen spinach

½ tablespoons of matcha

## Directions

Add all ingredients into a blender and combine until smooth.

Serve and enjoy!

## Recipe notes

Add in more liquid if you prefer a thinner smoothie and less for a thicker one. Use fewer avocados if you prefer a less creamy to greens ratio.

# Conclusion

We have come to the end of the book. Thank you for reading and congratulations for reading until the end.

If you found the book valuable, can you recommend it to others? One way to do that is to post a review on Amazon.

Please leave a review for this book on Amazon!

Thank you and good luck!

Printed in Great Britain
by Amazon